THE SUSTAINABLE KITCHEN:

Healthy Recipes for Long-Term Weight Loss

BY

STEPHANIE KNAPP

The Sustainable Kitchen is a book that is focused solely on the recipes and meal planning for a healthy and sustainable lifestyle. It is an extension of the previous book, with a more detailed approach on healthy eating habits and the recipes to support it. It is an excellent resource for anyone who wants to live a healthy lifestyle and maintain a healthy weight for life. This book is designed to help you make informed choices about what to eat while still enjoying your favorite foods in moderation. The recipes in this book are not only healthy but also delicious, making it easier to stick to your weight loss goals. So, let's dive in and start cooking up some delicious, healthy meals that will help you achieve your long-term weight loss goals!

TABLE OF CONTENTS

Introduction: Welcome to The Sustainable Kitchen

Welcome to The Sustainable Kitchen, a cookbook focused on providing you with healthy and sustainable recipes for long-term weight loss.

This book was written with you in mind, whether you are just starting your weight loss journey or looking for new ideas to spice up your healthy meal planning.

In today's fast-paced world, it can be challenging to maintain a healthy lifestyle. The rise of fast food and pre-packaged meals has made it easier than ever to fall into unhealthy eating habits. But with The Sustainable Kitchen, I hope to change that. I believe that healthy eating doesn't have to be bland or boring, and I'm excited to share my favorite recipes with you.

My goal is to provide you with healthy and delicious meals that are easy to prepare, whether you're a seasoned home cook or just getting started in the kitchen. I've included a variety of recipes, from hearty breakfast options to quick and easy snacks, satisfying main dishes, and indulgent desserts. I've also made sure to include options for all dietary preferences, including vegetarian and gluten-free.

In this book, you'll find more than just recipes. I've included tips on meal planning, grocery shopping, and cooking techniques to help you make the most of your time in the kitchen. I want to empower you to take control of your health and well-being by making healthy eating a sustainable lifestyle choice.

Thank you for joining me on this journey to a healthier, more sustainable life. Let's get cooking!

Chapter 1: The Importance of Nutrition in Sustainable Weight Loss

UNDERSTANDING THE ROLE OF MACRONUTRIENTS IN WEIGHT LOSS

Understanding the role of macronutrients in weight loss is a crucial step towards achieving and maintaining a healthy weight for life. In this chapter, we will explore the importance of macronutrients and how they can support your weight loss journey.

Macronutrients are the three primary sources of energy in our diet: carbohydrates, proteins, and fats. Each macronutrient has a unique role in our body, and an adequate balance of all three is essential for optimal health and weight loss.

Carbohydrates are the primary source of energy for our bodies. They are found in fruits, vegetables, grains, and legumes. Simple carbohydrates, such as those found in sugar and refined flour, are quickly digested and can lead to spikes in blood sugar levels. Complex carbohydrates, such as those found in whole grains, are slower to digest and can help stabilize blood sugar levels.

Protein is essential for building and repairing muscle tissue, and it is also a vital component of enzymes, hormones, and other body fluids. Sources of protein include meat, fish, poultry, beans, and tofu. Eating adequate protein can help prevent muscle loss during weight loss and may also help reduce appetite and promote satiety.

Fats are necessary for the absorption of certain vitamins and minerals, as well as for energy storage. Sources of healthy fats include nuts, seeds, avocados, and fatty fish. It is important to consume healthy fats in moderation, as they are more calorie-dense than carbohydrates and proteins.

When it comes to weight loss, it is important to create a calorie deficit, which means burning more calories than you consume. While all macronutrients contain calories, the ratio of carbohydrates, proteins, and fats in your diet can impact your weight loss progress.

Some popular weight loss diets, such as low-carb or high-protein diets, focus on manipulating the macronutrient ratios to achieve weight loss. However, it is important to remember that a sustainable and healthy weight loss plan should not rely on extreme restrictions or cutting out entire food groups.

Instead, focus on consuming a balanced diet that is rich in whole, nutrient-dense foods. Aim to fill your plate with colorful fruits and vegetables, lean proteins, healthy fats, and complex carbohydrates. This approach will help ensure that you are getting all the nutrients your body needs while also supporting weight loss.

In addition to the type of macronutrients you consume, the timing of your meals can also impact weight loss. Some people find that eating smaller, more frequent meals throughout the day helps keep hunger at bay and prevents overeating. Others may prefer larger, more satisfying meals with longer periods of fasting between meals.

Ultimately, the key to weight loss is finding what works best for your body and lifestyle. Experiment with different macronutrient ratios and meal timing strategies to find what feels most sustainable and effective for you.

It is also important to keep in mind that weight loss is not just about what you eat. Regular exercise, stress management, and adequate sleep are also crucial components of a healthy weight loss plan.

By understanding the role of macronutrients in weight loss and focusing on a balanced, nutrient-dense diet, you can set yourself up for sustainable weight loss success. Remember to listen to your body, stay consistent, and be patient with the process. With dedication and a healthy mindset, you can achieve and maintain a healthy weight for life.

NUTRIENT-DENSE FOODS FOR LONG-TERM SUCCESS

Eating a balanced and nutrient-dense diet is crucial for long-term success in achieving and maintaining a healthy weight. Nutrient-dense foods are those that are high in vitamins, minerals, and other beneficial nutrients, while also being relatively low in calories. These foods provide the body with the essential nutrients it needs to function optimally and support weight loss goals.

Here are some examples of nutrient-dense foods that can help you achieve long-term success in your weight loss journey:

Vegetables: Vegetables are some of the most nutrient-dense foods available. They are packed with vitamins, minerals, and antioxidants, and are also low in calories. Aim to include a variety of colorful vegetables in your diet, such as leafy greens, broccoli, peppers, and carrots.

Fruits: Fruits are another excellent source of essential nutrients, such as vitamins and fiber. They can also satisfy your sweet tooth without adding too many calories. Some nutrient-dense fruit options include berries, apples, and kiwi.

Lean proteins: Lean proteins such as chicken, turkey, fish, and tofu are excellent sources of essential amino acids, which are necessary for building and repairing tissues in the body. They can also help you feel full and satisfied, reducing the likelihood of overeating.

Whole grains: Whole grains such as brown rice, quinoa, and whole-grain bread are high in fiber and other essential nutrients. They can also help regulate blood sugar levels and keep you feeling full for longer.

Nuts and seeds: Nuts and seeds are packed with healthy fats, fiber, and other essential nutrients. They can help regulate blood sugar levels and keep you feeling full and satisfied.

It's important to note that just because a food is considered "healthy" doesn't mean it's automatically low in calories. Portion sizes and overall caloric intake still matter, even when choosing nutrient-dense foods. However, including these foods in your diet can help ensure you are getting the necessary nutrients to support your overall health and weight loss goals.

In addition to incorporating nutrient-dense foods into your diet, it's also important to make sure you are drinking enough water and limiting your intake of processed and high-calorie foods. By making these changes, you can create a sustainable and healthy diet that supports long-term success in achieving and maintaining a healthy weight.

TIPS FOR BUILDING A SUSTAINABLE MEAL PLAN

Building a sustainable meal plan is an essential component of long-term weight loss success. While many people focus on the latest diet fads or short-term fixes, the most effective way to lose weight and maintain a healthy lifestyle is to develop a sustainable approach to eating.

When it comes to building a sustainable meal plan, there are several key factors to consider. These include the types of foods you eat, the frequency and timing of your meals, and the overall structure of your diet. By focusing on these factors, you can create a meal plan that is healthy, satisfying, and sustainable over the long term.

Choose Nutrient-Dense Foods

The foundation of a sustainable meal plan is nutrient-dense foods. These are foods that are rich in nutrients like vitamins, minerals, fiber, and antioxidants, and are also relatively low in calories. Examples of nutrient-dense foods include fruits, vegetables, whole grains, lean proteins, and healthy fats.

When planning your meals, aim to incorporate a variety of nutrient-dense foods. This will ensure that you are getting a wide range of essential nutrients and will help keep you feeling full and satisfied.

Pay Attention to Portion Sizes

While the types of foods you eat are important, the amount of food you eat is also a key consideration. Paying attention to portion sizes can help you maintain a healthy weight and prevent overeating.

One way to control portion sizes is to use smaller plates and bowls. This can help you feel like you are eating a full meal while reducing the amount of food you consume. You can also use visual cues to help you estimate portion sizes. For example, a serving of protein should be about the size of a deck of cards, while a serving of vegetables should be about the size of your fist.

Plan Your Meals in Advance

Planning your meals in advance is an effective way to ensure that you are eating a balanced and nutrient-dense diet. By taking the time to plan your meals ahead of time, you can also save money and reduce food waste.

One way to plan your meals is to create a weekly meal plan. This can include a list of meals for each day of the week, along with a grocery list of the ingredients you will need. You can also prepare some meals in advance, such as by cooking a large batch of soup or chili at the beginning of the week and portioning it out for lunches.

Don't Skip Meals

Skipping meals is a common mistake that many people make when trying to lose weight. While it may seem like a good way to reduce your calorie intake, it can actually backfire and lead to overeating later in the day.

Instead of skipping meals, aim to eat smaller, more frequent meals throughout the day. This can help keep your blood sugar levels stable and prevent cravings and overeating.

Incorporate Treats in Moderation

Building a sustainable meal plan doesn't mean that you can't enjoy your favorite treats. In fact, allowing yourself to indulge in moderation can actually help you stick to your diet over the long term.

When incorporating treats into your meal plan, aim to do so in moderation. This might mean enjoying a small piece of chocolate after dinner or having a glass of wine with dinner once or twice a week.

By following these tips, you can build a sustainable meal plan that is healthy, satisfying, and effective for long-term weight loss success. Remember, the key to success is to make small, sustainable changes that you can stick with over time.

Chapter 2: Making Healthy Eating a Lifestyle

STRATEGIES FOR MEAL PLANNING AND PREPARATION

Meal planning and preparation are key components of any successful weight loss program. Having a plan in place can help you stay on track with your dietary goals, while also saving you time and money. Here are some strategies for effective meal planning and preparation:

Schedule a Weekly Planning Session: Set aside time each week to plan your meals for the upcoming week. This could be as simple as sitting down with a notepad and pen, or using a meal planning app to organize your recipes and grocery lists.

Choose Your Recipes: Choose a few recipes that you would like to make for the week, and write down the ingredients you will need. Look for recipes that are healthy and nutrient-dense, and that can be made in larger batches to save time.

Make a Grocery List: Based on the ingredients you will need for your chosen recipes, create a grocery list. This can help you stay focused at the store and avoid impulse purchases.

Shop Smart: When you get to the grocery store, stick to the items on your list. Avoid processed foods and pre-packaged meals, as they tend to be less healthy and more expensive.

Prep Ingredients in Advance: Once you have your groceries, take some time to prep your ingredients in advance. Chop vegetables, pre-cook grains, and marinate meat to save time during the week.

Batch Cook: If possible, make larger batches of your meals to have leftovers for the week. This can save you time and money, as well as prevent food waste.

Use Meal Prep Containers: Invest in some good-quality meal prep containers to store your prepared meals. This can help you stay organized, and makes it easier to take your meals with you on-the-go.

Try New Recipes: Experiment with new recipes and flavor combinations to keep your meals interesting and flavorful. This can help you stay motivated and engaged in your healthy eating plan.

Plan for Snacks: Don't forget to plan for healthy snacks as well. Pre-packaged snacks tend to be high in calories and low in nutrients, so consider making your own healthy snacks, such as fruit and nut bars or sliced veggies with hummus.

Be Flexible: Remember that meal planning is meant to be a tool to help you stay on track with your dietary goals. If something comes up during the week and you need to change your plans, don't stress about it. Use your meal plan as a guide, but allow yourself the flexibility to make changes as needed.

By implementing these strategies for meal planning and preparation, you can set yourself up for long-term success in your weight loss journey. Not only will you save time and money, but you will also be able to enjoy healthy, delicious meals that support your overall health and well-being.

MINDFUL EATING AND PORTION CONTROL

Mindful eating is a technique that encourages individuals to become more aware and present during meals. This can help to improve the relationship that an individual has with food and can also promote portion control, leading to a more balanced and nutrient-dense diet.

The first step in practicing mindful eating is to tune into your hunger and fullness cues. This means paying attention to your body and the physical sensations that you experience during meals. You should also take time to enjoy your food, focusing on the textures and flavors of each bite.

Another important aspect of mindful eating is to eliminate distractions during meals. This means turning off the TV and putting away your phone or computer. When you are focused on something else, you may not be aware of the amount of food you are consuming or the physical sensations of hunger and fullness.

Portion control is also an important component of mindful eating. Many people eat more than they need to simply because they are not paying attention to their body's cues. Some tips for practicing portion control include using smaller plates and bowls, measuring out portions of food, and avoiding eating straight from a package or container.

It's also important to be mindful of the types of food that you are consuming. Nutrient-dense foods should be a priority, as they provide the body with the vitamins, minerals, and other nutrients it needs to function properly. This includes plenty of fruits, vegetables, lean proteins, and whole grains. Processed and packaged foods, on the other hand, should be limited as much as possible.

By practicing mindful eating and portion control, individuals can improve their relationship with food and build a more sustainable and nutrient-dense diet over time.

NAVIGATING EATING OUT AND SOCIAL EVENTS

Eating out and social events can be a challenge when trying to maintain a healthy and sustainable diet. However, with a little planning and mindfulness, it's possible to make good choices and stick to your goals even when you're not in control of the menu.

Here are some tips for navigating eating out and social events:

- Plan ahead: Before you go out, check the menu or plan what you'll eat ahead of time. This can help you make healthier choices and avoid impulsively ordering something that doesn't align with your goals.

- Look for healthier options: Many restaurants now offer healthier options on their menus, so look for items that are grilled, baked, or steamed instead of fried. Choose lean protein sources like grilled chicken or fish, and opt for salads with dressing on the side.

- Watch your portions: Restaurant portions are often larger than what you'd eat at home, so be mindful of how much you're eating. Consider sharing an entree with a friend or taking half home for leftovers.

- Ask for modifications: Don't be afraid to ask for modifications to your meal, such as having sauce or dressing on the side, or substituting a side of vegetables for fries.

- Practice moderation: It's okay to indulge in a treat or a higher calorie meal once in a while, but don't let it become a regular habit. Practice moderation and make sure to balance indulgences with healthier choices the rest of the time.

- Be mindful of alcohol: Alcohol can be high in calories and can also lower your inhibitions and make it harder to stick to your goals. If you choose to drink, do so in moderation and consider lower calorie options like wine or a light beer.

- Bring a dish: If you're attending a social event, offer to bring a dish that aligns with your dietary goals. This ensures that there will be at least one healthy option available, and can also be a great conversation starter for others who are interested in healthy eating.

Remember, it's possible to make healthy choices even when you're not in control of the menu. By planning ahead, making mindful choices, and practicing moderation, you can still enjoy eating out and social events while sticking to your goals.

Chapter 3: Healthy and Delicious Breakfast Recipes

HIGH-PROTEIN BREAKFAST OPTIONS

High-protein breakfasts are an excellent way to start your day. They provide your body with the energy and nutrients it needs to function at its best, and they can help you feel fuller for longer, which can help with weight loss. In this section, we'll explore some delicious and nutritious high-protein breakfast options that are perfect for anyone looking to start their day off right.

- Greek Yogurt with Berries and Almonds: This is a quick and easy breakfast that is both high in protein and full of flavor. Simply spoon some Greek yogurt into a bowl and top with fresh berries and a handful of almonds. Greek yogurt is an excellent source of protein, with around 17 grams per cup, while berries are packed with antioxidants and vitamins. Almonds provide a good source of healthy fats and fiber.

- Veggie Omelet: Omelets are a classic breakfast dish that can be easily adapted to suit your tastes. To make a veggie omelet, simply whisk some eggs with a splash of milk and pour into a non-stick pan. Add your favorite veggies, such as bell peppers, spinach, and tomatoes, and cook until the eggs are set. Sprinkle with some cheese for an extra protein boost.

- Protein Pancakes: Who said pancakes can't be healthy? Protein pancakes are a delicious and nutritious option that can be enjoyed any day of the week. To make them, simply mix some protein powder with oats, almond milk, and an egg, and cook like regular pancakes. Serve with fresh fruit and a drizzle of honey for a tasty and filling breakfast.

- Chia Seed Pudding: Chia seeds are an excellent source of protein, with around 5 grams per ounce, and are also packed with fiber, omega-3 fatty acids, and other nutrients. To make chia seed pudding, simply mix some chia seeds with your favorite milk and sweetener, and let sit in the fridge overnight. In the morning, top with some fresh fruit and nuts for a delicious and satisfying breakfast.

- Breakfast Burrito: Breakfast burritos are a hearty and filling option that can be packed with protein and other nutrients. To make a breakfast burrito, scramble some eggs with veggies such as bell peppers, onions, and spinach. Add some black beans, avocado, and a sprinkle of cheese, and wrap in a whole-grain tortilla. This breakfast will keep you full for hours and is a great option for those on the go.

- Cottage Cheese and Fruit: Cottage cheese is a high-protein, low-fat dairy product that can be paired with almost any fruit for a delicious and nutritious breakfast. Simply top some cottage cheese with your favorite fruit, such as peaches, berries, or pineapple, and sprinkle with some nuts or granola for an extra crunch.

- Smoothie Bowl: Smoothie bowls are a great way to pack in a ton of nutrients and protein in one meal. To make a smoothie bowl, simply blend some frozen fruit, protein powder, and milk in a blender until smooth. Pour into a bowl and top with some granola, nuts, and fresh fruit for a filling and delicious breakfast.

In conclusion, there are many high-protein breakfast options to choose from, all of which can help keep you full and satisfied throughout the morning. Incorporating more protein into your diet can help with weight loss and overall health, and these breakfasts are a great way to start the day off on the right foot.

QUICK AND EASY BREAKFASTS FOR BUSY MORNINGS

Mornings can be hectic, and finding time to prepare and enjoy a healthy breakfast can be a challenge. However, skipping breakfast can leave you feeling hungry and lethargic, and may lead to overeating later in the day. The good news is that with a little planning and preparation, you can easily whip up a quick and healthy breakfast to start your day off right.

Here are some ideas for quick and easy breakfasts for busy mornings:

- Overnight oats: Combine rolled oats, milk or yogurt, and your favorite mix-ins in a jar or container and let it sit in the fridge overnight. In the morning, you'll have a delicious and nutritious breakfast that you can eat on the go.

- Smoothies: Blend together some fruit, yogurt or milk, and ice for a refreshing and filling breakfast smoothie. You can also add protein powder or nut butter for an extra boost of protein.

- Greek yogurt with fruit and granola: Greek yogurt is high in protein and can be topped with fresh fruit and granola for a quick and easy breakfast.

- Avocado toast: Mash up an avocado and spread it on whole grain toast for a filling and nutritious breakfast. You can also top it with a fried or scrambled egg for added protein.

- Breakfast burritos: Fill a tortilla with scrambled eggs, cheese, and veggies for a filling and portable breakfast.

- Energy balls: Make a batch of energy balls with oats, nut butter, and honey for a healthy and satisfying breakfast or snack.

- Egg muffins: Mix together eggs, veggies, and cheese and bake in a muffin tin for a quick and easy breakfast that you can make ahead of time and reheat throughout the week.

- Peanut butter banana toast: Spread peanut butter on whole grain toast and top with sliced banana for a simple and delicious breakfast.

- Cottage cheese with fruit: Cottage cheese is high in protein and can be topped with fresh fruit for a quick and easy breakfast.

- Breakfast bars: Make your own breakfast bars with oats, nuts, and dried fruit for a healthy and convenient breakfast option.

Incorporating healthy and quick breakfast options into your routine can set you up for success throughout the day. With a little creativity and planning, you can enjoy a nutritious and satisfying breakfast even on the busiest of mornings.

MEAL PREP IDEAS FOR BREAKFAST

In this section, we will discuss some meal prep ideas for breakfast that will save you time and ensure you have a healthy breakfast every day.

- Overnight Oats: This is a classic breakfast meal prep idea that is easy to make and can be customized to your liking. Simply mix oats, milk, yogurt, and your favorite toppings like fruit, nuts, and seeds in a jar or container, and leave it in the fridge overnight. In the morning, you will have a delicious and nutritious breakfast waiting for you.

- Egg Muffins: These are another easy breakfast meal prep idea that can be made ahead of time and stored in the fridge or freezer. Simply whisk eggs with your favorite veggies, cheese, and spices, pour the mixture into muffin cups, and bake in the oven until cooked through. You can make a batch of these on the weekend and enjoy them throughout the week.

- Smoothie Packs: Smoothies are a great way to get a healthy breakfast in a hurry, but they can be time-consuming to make every morning. To save time, you can prepare smoothie packs ahead of time by portioning out your favorite fruits, veggies, and protein powders into ziplock bags or containers. When you're ready to make a smoothie, simply blend the contents of the pack with milk or water.

- Yogurt Parfaits: Yogurt parfaits are a simple and delicious breakfast option that can be made in advance. Layer Greek yogurt, fruit, and granola in a jar or container, and store it in the fridge until you're ready to eat. You can also add nuts or seeds for an extra crunch.

- Breakfast Burritos: If you're a fan of savory breakfasts, breakfast burritos are a great option. Make a big batch of scrambled eggs, black beans, and your favorite veggies, and wrap them in whole-grain tortillas. You can then freeze the burritos and reheat them in the microwave for a quick breakfast on the go.

Here are some more meal prep ideas for breakfast:

Breakfast burritos: Make a big batch of scrambled eggs, sautéed veggies, and beans, then wrap in a tortilla for an easy on-the-go breakfast.

- Greek yogurt bowls: Mix plain Greek yogurt with your favorite toppings such as fruit, nuts, and granola for a satisfying and high-protein breakfast.

- Chia pudding: Combine chia seeds with milk, sweetener, and flavorings such as vanilla or cocoa powder, and let it sit in the fridge overnight. In the morning, add your favorite toppings such as fruit and nuts.

- Quiche: Make a big batch of crustless quiche with eggs, vegetables, and cheese for a protein-packed breakfast that can be easily reheated throughout the week.

- Breakfast sandwiches: Make a batch of English muffins or bagels with eggs, cheese, and turkey sausage for a delicious and filling breakfast that can be easily reheated.

- Pancakes or waffles: Make a big batch of pancakes or waffles on the weekend, then freeze them in individual portions for an easy breakfast throughout the week.

- Breakfast bars: Make your own breakfast bars with wholesome ingredients such as oats, nuts, and dried fruit for a quick and easy breakfast on the go.

These are just a few meal prep ideas for breakfast that can help you save time and eat healthy. With a little bit of planning and preparation, you can enjoy a nutritious breakfast every day without sacrificing your busy schedule.

Chapter 4: Satisfying and Nutritious Lunch Recipes

FRESH AND FILLING SALAD IDEAS
Here are 40 fresh and filling salad ideas:

1. Classic Cobb Salad
2. Caprese Salad
3. Greek Salad
4. Caesar Salad
5. Strawberry Spinach Salad
6. Chicken Caesar Salad
7. Southwest Salad
8. Tuna Salad
9. Quinoa Salad
10. Waldorf Salad
11. Grilled Chicken Salad
12. Broccoli Salad
13. Chef Salad
14. Asian Slaw
15. Beet Salad
16. Taco Salad
17. Nicoise Salad
18. Mediterranean Salad
19. Kale Caesar Salad
20. Spinach and Feta Salad
21. Chicken Caprese Salad
22. Watermelon and Feta Salad
23. Antipasto Salad
24. Steak Salad
25. Shrimp Salad
26. Egg Salad

27. Roasted Butternut Squash Salad
28. Cobb Salad Wraps
29. Chicken and Avocado Salad
30. Chicken and Bacon Salad
31. Strawberry and Goat Cheese Salad
32. Shrimp and Avocado Salad
33. Grilled Halloumi Salad
34. Grilled Peach Salad
35. Broccoli Slaw
36. Tomato and Mozzarella Salad
37. Fajita Salad
38. Asian Chicken Salad
39. Roasted Veggie Salad
40. Summer Fruit Salad

These salads are all fresh, filling, and easy to make. They can be customized to suit your preferences and dietary needs, and can be enjoyed as a main dish or a side dish.

EASY LUNCH OPTIONS FOR WORK OR SCHOOL

When it comes to healthy eating and weight loss, lunch is an important meal that shouldn't be overlooked. Unfortunately, with busy work schedules or the rush of school, it can be difficult to find time to prepare a nutritious lunch. The good news is that with a little planning and preparation, there are plenty of easy and healthy lunch options that can be made ahead of time and brought to work or school.

- Mason Jar Salads: Mason jar salads are a quick and easy way to prepare a nutritious and filling lunch. Simply layer your favorite salad ingredients in a jar and store in the fridge. When it's time for lunch, just shake the jar and enjoy. Some good options for layering include leafy greens, protein (such as chicken or tofu), nuts or seeds, and a vinaigrette dressing.

- Veggie Wraps: Wraps are a great way to get in your daily dose of veggies. Simply wrap your favorite veggies (such as lettuce, tomato, cucumber, and avocado) in a whole wheat or gluten-free wrap, and top with a protein source (such as grilled chicken or chickpeas) and a light dressing.

- Quinoa Bowls: Quinoa bowls are a filling and nutrient-dense lunch option that can be customized to your liking. Cook quinoa according to the package directions, and top with your favorite veggies (such as roasted sweet potato, sautéed spinach, and roasted red pepper), protein (such as grilled chicken or tempeh), and a healthy fat (such as avocado).

- Soup: Soup is a great lunch option that can be made ahead of time and stored in the fridge or freezer. Try making a large batch of your favorite vegetable soup or chili, and portion it out for a week's worth of lunches.

- Bento Boxes: Bento boxes are a fun and creative way to pack a nutritious lunch. Simply divide a container into compartments and fill with your favorite veggies, protein (such as sliced deli meat or hard-boiled eggs), fruit, and a healthy fat (such as nuts or hummus).

With these easy and healthy lunch options, you can stay on track with your weight loss goals while still enjoying a delicious and satisfying meal. Just remember to plan ahead, prep your meals in advance, and make sure to pack plenty of fresh veggies and protein to keep you full and energized throughout the day.

SOUPS AND STEWS FOR A COZY AND HEALTHY MEAL

Soups and stews are comforting and delicious meals that are perfect for cold weather. They are also a great way to pack in a lot of nutritious ingredients in a single dish. Here are 20 soups and stews that are both cozy and healthy:

1) Chicken Noodle Soup: This classic soup is packed with vegetables, tender chicken, and noodles in a savory broth.

2) Tomato Soup: A simple yet satisfying soup made with ripe tomatoes and fresh herbs.

3) Lentil Soup: A hearty soup made with protein-rich lentils and a variety of vegetables and spices.

4) Butternut Squash Soup: A creamy and flavorful soup made with roasted butternut squash and a touch of cream.

5) Minestrone Soup: A vegetable-packed soup with beans, pasta, and a flavorful tomato broth.

6) Beef Stew: A comforting stew made with tender beef, vegetables, and a rich tomato and wine broth.

7) Vegetable Soup: A light and healthy soup made with a variety of fresh vegetables and a savory broth.

8) Potato Soup: A creamy and satisfying soup made with potatoes, cheese, and bacon.

9) Black Bean Soup: A spicy and flavorful soup made with black beans, vegetables, and spices.

10)   Clam Chowder: A creamy and hearty soup made with fresh clams, potatoes, and cream.

11)   Split Pea Soup: A flavorful and satisfying soup made with split peas, ham, and vegetables.

12)   White Bean and Kale Soup: A hearty and nutritious soup made with white beans, kale, and vegetables.

13)   Chicken and Dumplings: A comforting soup made with tender chicken, fluffy dumplings, and a savory broth.

14)   Corn Chowder: A creamy and comforting soup made with fresh corn, potatoes, and cream.

15)   Gazpacho: A refreshing and healthy cold soup made with fresh vegetables, olive oil, and vinegar.

16)   French Onion Soup: A rich and flavorful soup made with caramelized onions, beef broth, and crusty bread.

17)   Chicken Tortilla Soup: A spicy and flavorful soup made with tender chicken, vegetables, and crunchy tortilla strips.

18)   Beef and Barley Soup: A comforting and hearty soup made with tender beef, vegetables, and barley.

19)   Cabbage Soup: A healthy and light soup made with cabbage, vegetables, and a savory broth.

20)   Chili: A spicy and flavorful stew made with ground beef, beans, and spices.

These soups and stews are perfect for a cozy and nutritious meal that will keep you warm and satisfied. Try them out and experiment with different flavors and ingredients to find your favorite combinations.

HIGH-PROTEIN AND LOW-CARB OPTIONS

High-protein and low-carb options are great for those looking to lose weight, build muscle, or just maintain a healthy lifestyle. These types of meals can help you feel full and satisfied while also providing your body with the nutrients it needs to function properly.

Some examples of high-protein and low-carb meals include grilled chicken with roasted vegetables, a spinach salad with hard-boiled eggs and avocado, or a stir-fry with lean beef and a variety of colorful vegetables. Other options include low-carb wraps with turkey or chicken, omelets with veggies and cheese, and grilled fish with a side of steamed vegetables.

To ensure that your meals are both high in protein and low in carbs, focus on lean protein sources such as chicken, turkey, fish, and tofu, and incorporate plenty of non-starchy vegetables such as spinach, kale, broccoli, and peppers. You can also include healthy fats such as nuts, seeds, and avocado to help keep you full and satisfied.

When planning your high-protein and low-carb meals, it's important to keep in mind your personal dietary needs and goals. If you're trying to lose weight, it's important to focus on portion control and create a calorie deficit. However, if you're looking to build muscle, you may need to increase your overall calorie intake and focus on consuming enough protein to support muscle growth.

Overall, high-protein and low-carb meals can be a great addition to a healthy, balanced diet. By incorporating a variety of nutrient-dense foods, you can support your overall health and wellbeing while also achieving your weight loss or muscle-building goals.

VEGETARIAN AND VEGAN DINNERS

If you are looking for vegetarian and vegan dinner ideas, we have got you covered. In this section, we will share 20 delicious and nutritious vegetarian and vegan dinners that will satisfy your taste buds and keep you feeling full and energized.

- Vegan Buddha Bowl: This bowl is packed with plant-based protein, fiber, and healthy fats. It features brown rice, roasted chickpeas, avocado, roasted vegetables, and a creamy tahini dressing.

- Cauliflower Fried Rice: This low-carb, vegetarian version of fried rice uses grated cauliflower instead of rice. It is packed with vegetables, eggs, and a flavorful sauce.

- Lentil Shepherd's Pie: This vegan version of the classic comfort food is made with lentils, vegetables, and topped with creamy mashed potatoes.

- Chickpea Curry: This spicy, flavorful curry is made with chickpeas, vegetables, and coconut milk. It is served over brown rice or quinoa.

- Stuffed Peppers: These colorful bell peppers are filled with a mix of rice, vegetables, and protein (such as tofu or beans).

- Vegan Chili: This hearty chili is made with beans, vegetables, and spices. It is served with your choice of toppings, such as avocado, cilantro, or vegan cheese.

- Ratatouille: This classic French dish is made with eggplant, zucchini, tomatoes, and bell peppers. It can be served as a side dish or as a main course with crusty bread.

- Spaghetti Squash with Tomato Sauce: This low-carb, vegetarian version of spaghetti features roasted spaghetti squash and a flavorful tomato sauce.

- Veggie Burgers: These plant-based burgers are made with a mix of beans, grains, and vegetables. They can be served with your choice of toppings, such as avocado, lettuce, and tomato.

- Tofu Stir-Fry: This quick and easy stir-fry features tofu, vegetables, and a flavorful sauce. It can be served over rice or noodles.

- Vegan Lasagna: This hearty lasagna is made with layers of pasta, vegetables, and a creamy cashew cheese sauce.

- Quinoa Stuffed Portobello Mushrooms: These meaty Portobello mushrooms are filled with a mix of quinoa, vegetables, and spices.

- Vegan Mac and Cheese: This creamy and comforting mac and cheese is made with a cashew cheese sauce.

- Chickpea and Spinach Curry: This vegan curry is made with chickpeas, spinach, and spices. It is served over brown rice or quinoa.

- Falafel: These crispy, flavorful chickpea patties are served with pita bread and a tahini sauce.

- Vegan Pad Thai: This classic Thai dish is made with rice noodles, vegetables, and tofu. It is served with a tangy and spicy sauce.

- Lentil Meatballs: These vegetarian meatballs are made with lentils, breadcrumbs, and spices. They can be served with marinara sauce and spaghetti.

- Vegan Fajitas: These colorful fajitas are made with bell peppers, onions, and a protein of your choice (such as tofu or beans). They are served with tortillas and your choice of toppings.

- Mushroom Stroganoff: This vegetarian version of the classic Russian dish is made with mushrooms, sour cream, and egg noodles.

- Vegan Pizza: This plant-based pizza can be topped with your choice of vegetables, vegan cheese, and a flavorful tomato sauce.

COMFORT FOOD MADE HEALTHY

When it comes to comfort food, many people have fond memories of their favorite meals from childhood or special occasions. However, these dishes are often high in calories, unhealthy fats, and refined carbohydrates that can sabotage weight loss efforts.

But the good news is that you don't have to give up your favorite comfort foods to maintain a healthy weight. With a few simple swaps and substitutions, you can make your favorite dishes healthier and more nutritious.

One of the keys to making comfort food healthier is to use whole, unprocessed ingredients whenever possible. For example, instead of using white pasta or rice, opt for whole-grain versions, which provide more fiber and nutrients.

Another way to lighten up comfort food is to use leaner proteins, such as skinless chicken breast or lean ground turkey, instead of fatty cuts of meat. You can also experiment with vegetarian and plant-based sources of protein, such as tofu, tempeh, beans, and lentils.

In addition to swapping ingredients, you can also modify the cooking method to make comfort food healthier. For example, instead of deep-frying chicken or fish, try baking, grilling, or broiling it instead. You can also use non-stick cooking spray or a small amount of healthy oil, such as olive or avocado oil, instead of butter or lard.

Another way to boost the nutritional value of comfort food is to add more vegetables. This not only adds more nutrients and fiber but also helps to bulk up the dish, making it more filling and satisfying. You can add vegetables to dishes in a variety of ways, such as using them as a base for stews, casseroles, or soups, or adding them as a side dish or topping.

Here are some examples of comfort foods that can be made healthier with simple swaps and modifications:

- Macaroni and cheese: Use whole-grain pasta, low-fat cheese, and add steamed broccoli or cauliflower for a boost of nutrients.

- Meatloaf: Use lean ground turkey or beef, add chopped vegetables like carrots and celery, and use whole-grain breadcrumbs.

- Fried chicken: Use skinless chicken breast, coat in whole-grain breadcrumbs, and bake or grill instead of frying.

- Pizza: Use a whole-grain crust, low-fat cheese, and add plenty of vegetables like bell peppers, mushrooms, and spinach.

- Chili: Use lean ground turkey or beef, add plenty of beans and vegetables, and top with a dollop of low-fat sour cream or Greek yogurt.

By making these simple swaps and modifications, you can enjoy your favorite comfort foods without sacrificing your health or weight loss goals. Not only will your body thank you, but you'll also feel good about indulging in these nostalgic and delicious dishes.

Chapter 6: Delicious and Nutritious Snack Recipes

HOMEMADE SNACKS TO SATISFY CRAVINGS

Making homemade snacks can be a great way to satisfy cravings while still sticking to a healthy diet. Here are some ideas for homemade snacks that are both delicious and nutritious:

- Roasted chickpeas: Roasting chickpeas with spices such as cumin, paprika, and garlic powder can create a crunchy and savory snack.

- Trail mix: Mixing together nuts, seeds, and dried fruit can create a satisfying and portable snack.

- Energy balls: Mixing together ingredients such as dates, nuts, and coconut flakes can create a sweet and nutritious snack that can be eaten on the go.

- Greek yogurt with fruit and honey: Mixing together Greek yogurt with fresh fruit and a drizzle of honey can create a sweet and creamy snack that is high in protein.

- Baked sweet potato fries: Slicing sweet potatoes into thin fries and baking them in the oven with a drizzle of olive oil and spices can create a healthier alternative to regular french fries.

- Homemade popcorn: Making popcorn on the stove with a drizzle of olive oil and spices such as nutritional yeast can create a delicious and low-calorie snack.

- Veggie sticks with hummus: Cutting up fresh veggies such as carrots, cucumbers, and bell peppers and dipping them in homemade hummus can create a crunchy and satisfying snack.

- Dark chocolate-covered almonds: Melting dark chocolate and dipping almonds in it can create a sweet and indulgent snack that is high in protein and healthy fats.

- Homemade granola bars: Mixing together oats, nuts, and dried fruit with a binder such as peanut butter can create a healthy and filling snack that can be eaten on the go.

- Fresh fruit with nut butter: Slicing up fresh fruit and spreading nut butter on top can create a sweet and filling snack that is high in protein and healthy fats.

LOW-CALORIE OPTIONS FOR ON-THE-GO

When you're constantly on the go, it can be difficult to find healthy, low-caloric options that you can grab and take with you. But with a little bit of planning and preparation, you can easily have a variety of tasty and nutritious snacks and meals to keep you going throughout the day.

Here are some low-calorie options for on-the-go:

- Fresh fruit: Fruit is a great snack to take with you on-the-go because it's portable and requires no preparation. Choose fruits that are easy to eat on the go, like bananas, apples, or grapes.

- Raw vegetables: Raw vegetables like carrots, celery, and cucumbers are low in calories and high in fiber, making them a perfect snack for those watching their weight.

- Greek yogurt: Greek yogurt is a great source of protein and can be a satisfying snack on its own or combined with fruit or nuts.

- Hard-boiled eggs: Hard-boiled eggs are a great source of protein and can be a filling and satisfying snack or meal on-the-go.

- Rice cakes with nut butter: Rice cakes are a low-calorie, crunchy snack that can be a satisfying treat when paired with nut butter, which is a great source of healthy fats and protein.

- Popcorn: Popcorn is a low-calorie snack that can be a satisfying treat when air-popped and lightly salted.

- Trail mix: Make your own trail mix with a mix of nuts, seeds, and dried fruit for a healthy and filling snack.

- Smoothies: Smoothies are a great way to pack in lots of nutrients on-the-go. Use low-calorie fruits and vegetables like berries, spinach, and kale, and add in a source of protein like Greek yogurt or protein powder.

By having a variety of these low-calorie options on hand, you'll be able to stay satisfied and energized throughout the day, even when you're on-the-go.

SNACKS FOR PRE- AND POST-WORKOUT FUEL

Snacks are an essential part of any workout regimen. Whether you're looking to fuel up before a workout or recover after one, the right snack can help you perform your best and see the best results. When it comes to pre-workout snacks, you want something that will give you the energy and endurance you need to power through your workout. And for post-workout snacks, you need something that will help your body recover, rebuild and refuel.

Here are some healthy and delicious snack ideas for pre- and post-workout fuel:

- Apple slices with almond butter: This classic combo is packed with fiber, protein, and healthy fats, making it a great option for pre- and post-workout fuel.

- Greek yogurt with berries: Greek yogurt is high in protein and low in fat, while berries are full of antioxidants and nutrients. Together, they make a great post-workout snack.

- Hard-boiled eggs: Hard-boiled eggs are a great source of protein, making them a perfect pre-workout snack. They are also easy to take on the go.

- Protein smoothie: Blend together a scoop of protein powder, some frozen fruit, and a handful of spinach for a quick and easy post-workout snack.

- Hummus and veggies: Hummus is a great source of protein and healthy fats, while veggies are packed with nutrients. Together, they make a great pre- or post-workout snack.

- Trail mix: Mix together some nuts, seeds, and dried fruit for a portable and filling snack that is perfect for pre-workout fuel.

- Turkey roll-ups: Wrap slices of turkey around a piece of cheese or a dollop of hummus for a protein-packed snack that is perfect for post-workout recovery.

Remember, snacks are an important part of your overall nutrition plan. Make sure to choose snacks that are healthy, nutrient-dense, and satisfying to help you reach your fitness goals.

HEALTHY DESSERTS AND SWEET TREATS

Healthy desserts and sweet treats can be a great way to satisfy your sweet tooth without compromising your health goals. By using nutrient-dense ingredients and natural sweeteners, you can create delicious and satisfying desserts that are also good for you. Here are some ideas for healthy desserts and sweet treats:

- Fruit-based desserts: Fresh or frozen fruits can be turned into delicious desserts with a little creativity. Some ideas include fruit salads, grilled fruit skewers, fruit sorbets, and fruit smoothies.

- Dark chocolate: Dark chocolate is rich in antioxidants and can be a healthy treat in moderation. Look for high-quality dark chocolate with at least 70% cocoa solids.

- Healthy baking: You can make your favorite baked goods healthier by using whole grain flour, natural sweeteners like honey or maple syrup, and adding nutrient-dense ingredients like nuts, seeds, or fruit.

- Chia pudding: Chia seeds are high in fiber and omega-3 fatty acids, and can be used to create a creamy and satisfying pudding. Mix chia seeds with milk, sweetener, and flavorings like vanilla or cocoa powder, and let it sit in the fridge overnight.

- Yogurt parfaits: Layer yogurt, fruit, and nuts or granola for a healthy and satisfying dessert or snack.

- Frozen treats: You can make your own healthy frozen treats by blending frozen fruit, yogurt, and other ingredients like honey or cocoa powder, and freezing the mixture in popsicle molds.

- Nut butter snacks: Nut butters like peanut butter, almond butter, or cashew butter can be a satisfying and healthy snack when paired with fruit or whole grain crackers.

By incorporating these healthy dessert and sweet treat options into your diet, you can satisfy your cravings without sacrificing your health goals. Remember to enjoy these treats in moderation and balance them with a diet rich in whole, nutrient-dense foods.

TIPS FOR NAVIGATING HOLIDAY MEALS AND EVENTS

Navigating holiday meals and events can be challenging when you're trying to maintain a healthy lifestyle. However, it's important to remember that you can still enjoy the festivities while sticking to your goals. Here are some solid tips for navigating holiday meals and events:

1) Plan ahead: Before attending a holiday meal or event, plan what you're going to eat and how much you'll indulge. Stick to your plan to avoid overindulging in unhealthy options.

2) Bring your own dish: Consider bringing a healthy dish to share. This ensures that there will be at least one healthy option available, and it's also a great way to introduce your friends and family to new and healthy foods.

3) Fill up on vegetables: Look for vegetable-based dishes and fill up on those before moving on to heavier or more indulgent dishes.

4) Practice mindful eating: Take your time when eating and savor every bite. This will not only help you enjoy your food more, but it will also help you tune in to your body's hunger and fullness signals.

5) Stay hydrated: Drinking plenty of water throughout the day can help you stay hydrated and keep you feeling full.

6) Avoid temptation: If there are certain foods that are particularly tempting to you, try to avoid them altogether. This will help you stay on track and avoid unnecessary calories.

7) Enjoy in moderation: It's okay to indulge in your favorite holiday treats, but do so in moderation. Practice portion control and savor every bite.

By following these tips, you can enjoy holiday meals and events while still staying on track with your healthy lifestyle.

CELEBRATING PROGRESS WITH HEALTHY INDULGENCES

Conclusion: Sustainable Weight Loss for Life

Celebrating progress with healthy indulgences is a crucial part of maintaining a sustainable weight loss plan. The idea of indulging in foods that you enjoy can be tempting, but it can also cause guilt and disrupt your progress. Fortunately, there are plenty of healthy indulgences that you can enjoy without feeling guilty.

One way to celebrate your progress is by treating yourself to a healthy dessert. Instead of indulging in a high-calorie cake or pie, opt for a healthier alternative such as fresh fruit, Greek yogurt, or a small serving of dark chocolate. These treats are not only delicious but also rich in nutrients that your body needs.

Another way to celebrate your progress is by treating yourself to a fun and active outing. You can go for a hike, take a dance class, or try a new sport. These activities not only provide a great workout but also help you unwind and relieve stress. You can also invite friends and family to join you for a group outing, which can be a great way to celebrate your progress and bond with loved ones.

It's also important to remember that celebrating progress doesn't always have to be about food or physical activity. You can treat yourself to a spa day, take a weekend getaway, or simply spend time doing something that you love. These activities can help you relax and recharge, which is crucial for maintaining a healthy and sustainable lifestyle.

Ultimately, the key to celebrating progress with healthy indulgences is finding a balance between indulging in the things you love and maintaining your healthy habits. By incorporating these tips into your routine, you can celebrate your progress without derailing your weight loss journey.

The Sustainable Fat Loss Solution: Achieving and Maintaining a Healthy Weight for Life

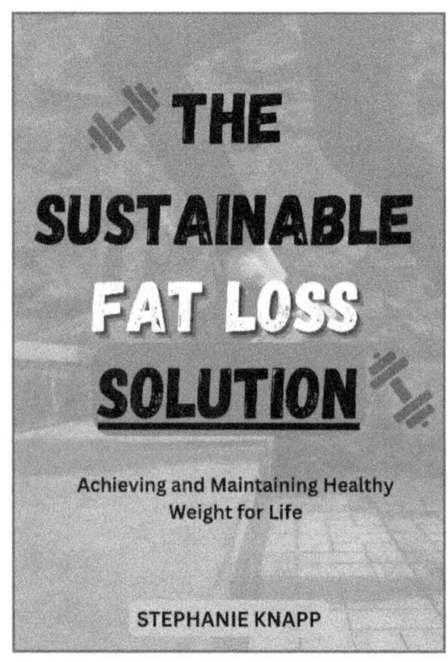

You can get the kindle version of this book for free by ;

1. Leaving a positive review on " THE SUSTAINABLE KITCHEN" 'S Amazon kindle page

2. Purchasing the Kindle version of "THE SUSTAINABLE KITCHEN"

Send proof to our agent via this link [www.tinyurl.com/Stephanie-knapp-Purchase-Proof] and receive your copy immediately!!!